ADDICTION MANAGEMENT

THE CONTROL OF CRAVING

A Guide for Self, Family, and Friends

Charles F Clark, MD, MPH, retired

Copyright: February 11, 2024
ISBN: 979832123967
Imprint: Independently published

Editor: Don Yannicito

In memory of my wife,
   Carol Wells McCoy Clark
      June 17, 1938 - October 16, 2020

Other books by the author:
AIDS and the Arrows of Pestilence
Growing Magic Mushrooms (with Martha Friedrich)
Colorado Legal Psychedelics: Psilocybin, Psilocin, DMT, Mescaline and Ibogaine

Table of Contents

SECTION 3: THE CONTROL OF CHRONIC PAIN

Preface

Control of craving is the key to managing addictions.
Addictions   are normal behavior gone awry. Prior to
1900, no addicting substances were banned or illegal in
the United States. Cocaine was an ingredient in
Coca-Cola. Heroin and cocaine were available for sale in
the Sears and Roebuck catalog along with a syringe to
use for their injection. Morphine was a routine ingredient
in cough syrups and antidiarrheal medications. All sorts of
remedies for aches and pains contained heroin or
morphine. None of these medications required a
prescription. Neither marijuana nor tobacco were
regulated.

Despite this widespread easy availability of inexpensive
substances that we now breathlessly call dangerous
drugs, the country was not falling apart and crime was not
rampant. There were no criminal gangs shooting each
other for control over the distribution of these substances.
There were addicts, especially to alcohol, and there were
associated significant social problems. Then as now,
alcohol was by far the biggest social problem. There were
many morphine addicts, generally people with chronic
pain problems. After the Civil War there were so many
wounded soldiers addicted to morphine that it was called
the "soldier's disease".

All that changed in 1914 when for political, not medical reasons, addicting substances began to be regulated and then outlawed. In 1970, again for political, not medical reasons, America began a war on drugs, filling our prisons and creating thousands of law enforcement jobs. Addicts are withdrawn from these substances over and over again through incarceration and abstinence treatment. It has had little lasting effect. Those efforts have not made us safer or healthier.

The problem is that we have not addressed the craving that the addict experiences for the drug. This book suggests possible solutions.

INTRODUCTION

Humans manage to addict themselves to many different substances which have a startling variety of effects. Some addictive drugs wake you up and increase your concentration. Others put you to sleep. Some decrease your anxiety. Another, alcohol, lubricates social interaction and decreases social control. Some reduce the awareness of pain. These are amazingly different, even contradictory, drug experiences to which a small number of people will become so attached that in the pursuit of that special feeling they will damage their health, and sometimes abandon their families or even fall into homelessness.

Most people use these substances occasionally, intermittently or modestly, and never become addicted. They do not develop a craving for the substances. Most people who become addicted continue to function as responsible citizens although their relationships and performance suffer. The term addictive personality is sometimes applied to a person who is addicted to multiple drugs or who becomes addicted to one drug after another. There is no evidence for such a personality type. Addiction occurs in all kinds of people in all sorts of circumstances and some are unlucky enough to be easily addicted to multiple substances.

Only one of these addicting substances, alcohol, causes damage to nerves in the brain and elsewhere. None of the others cause harm to the nervous system. All of the others perform their action by tweaking receptors on neurons in the brain and elsewhere so that the neurons fire at a faster or slower rate. Stop the addicting substance, and with the passage of some time, the neurons go back to working normally. However, lurking somewhere in the brains of addicts is a feeling that misses the drug immensely. This is the craving that drives the addict back to using the drug. It has many variations and permutations and can be triggered by all sorts of sights, smells, and situations. It is the unrelenting craving that makes a person an addict.

Withdrawal from alcohol and opiates can cause terrible withdrawal symptoms which can be life threatening. Once that process is over, it is the craving that drives the person back to use. Many antidepressant medications, for example venlafaxine, trade name Effexor, have severe withdrawal symptoms, but once withdrawal is completed, there is no craving for the drug. This is true of some other drugs as well. Withdrawal symptoms do not determine which drugs are addicting. Craving determines addiction.

Addicting drugs can then be defined as substances which cause craving in a small percentage of the population once they have had adequate exposure. Treatment of addiction must therefore address craving. The success of treatments, regardless of their widely differing psychological and medication approaches, will be determined by how effectively they suppress or control craving.

There appears to be a relationship between addiction to drugs (specific chemicals) and behavior (gambling and excessive eating). The diabetic treatment drugs, semaglutide (trade names Ozempic and Wegovy) and dulaglutide (trade name Trulicity) decrease appetite (food craving) leading to weight loss. They are now officially approved for this indication. In addition, in about 50% of people, they decrease craving for alcohol and tobacco! In studies with rats they also decrease consumption of opiates and stimulants (cocaine and amphetamines).

This book discusses the nine major categories of addictions. Many readers will have an interest only in the addiction(s) to which they, a family member, or friend, are suffering. It is only necessary to read chapters 1 and 2, then the chapter on the addiction of interest, and chapter 10 to understand the problem. For the potential solution, read the rest of the book which addresses how to control craving for addicting substances by using available medications or dietary substances.

SECTION 1: THE ADDICTIONS

CHAPTER 1

THE ADDICTIONS PROBLEM

Drug addiction is a thorn in the side of American society. The total federal spending on drug enforcement in 2022 was 41 billion dollars. The Drug Enforcement Administration employs 10,000 people working in 334 offices in the United States and around the world. There has been a 50 year failed effort to stem the flow of illegal drugs into the United States. Consumer demand by non-addicted and addicted persons drives the importation.

About 83,000 Americans die every year from opiate overdoses, and many more careers and families are devastated. Stimulant addiction (cocaine and amphetamines) kills only about 20,000 persons each year, but is terribly disruptive to a much larger number of families and to society. Alcohol, a legal drug, kills even more than the opiates and stimulants, and wrecks far more careers and families. Approximately one in ten American adults is addicted to alcohol which in medical terminology is called Alcohol Use Disorder. A failed attempt at making alcohol illegal from 1920 to 1933 demonstrated the futility of attempting to reduce a drug's effect on society by banning its availability. Currently 180,000 Americans die each year as a result of alcohol addiction. That is twice as many as die from opiates. Tobacco kills even more than all the other drugs combined, about 480,000 each year which includes 41,000 dying from exposure to secondhand smoke. For a sense of the impact of these combined 700,000 drug deaths on society, compare it to cancer, which kills 608,000 yearly and heart disease, which kills 685,000 Americans each year.

Often unmentioned is that the most widely used addicting drug in America and the world is caffeine, the active ingredient in coffee and tea and many other drinks including Coca-Cola. It is not considered a problem as there are almost no health consequences even to very heavy use, and it does not cause socially unacceptable behavior. Tobacco used to be in the same category as caffeine until it was noticed that those smoking regularly were dying at a high rate from lung cancer, heart disease and emphysema. If you are a regular coffee or tea drinker, the physical and emotional discomfort in the morning are the symptoms of withdrawal from caffeine. Those symptoms are relieved by a morning cup of coffee or tea just as opiate withdrawal is relieved by an injection of heroin.

CHAPTER 2

WHY MEDICAL TREATMENT IS RARELY SUCCESSFUL

Addictions are not like other human diseases. They don't just happen to us. We humans have had to seek out substances that alter our state of mind in order to make ourselves subject to drug addictions. Addictions are not ancient human diseases like arthritis, cancer, heart disease, or diabetes. They aren't diseases that infect us like tuberculosis, malaria, measles, or influenza. Humans had to go out into the world to find special substances, process them into easily ingested forms, and take them in sufficient quantities to alter the perception of reality.

You have to take the potentially addictive substance persistently enough to develop a craving for it. Addiction, then, in a peculiar sense, is a voluntary disease. You must make significant efforts to acquire the disease, and then you must persist in your efforts to maintain the disease.

What is remarkable is that most human beings who seek out and use the addicting substances for appropriate reasons such as pain or to stay awake or for entertainment, do not find them to be attractive enough to use on a regular basis, and never become addicted! Most American adults have used opiates either secondary to an accident or surgery or for entertainment. Less than 1% subsequently use opiates so repeatedly as to become addicted. About 80 percent of

American adults have tried alcohol, but only 10 percent are addicted. Tobacco is the most addictive substance known to humans. Tobacco addiction rates are as high as 40 percent among those who use it multiple times.

Many people use these potentially addicting substances occasionally, sporadically, in varying amounts and for a multitude of reasons, and with the exception of tobacco, never become addicted. They may enjoy the drug or drugs, use them for fun or to treat pain, and never are inclined to use them regularly to the point of addiction. The amphetamines and cocaine may be used by most people to improve short term performance and wakefulness or for fun without creating addiction. Modern combat forces would be at a terrible disadvantage if deprived of these stimulants. Soldiers and airmen are routinely given stimulants to stay awake and to maintain an aggressive attitude. This massive use of stimulants began in World War I with cocaine, and then amphetamines, and continues to the present day in all armies.

So why do many users of tobacco become addicted? Why do a modest number of alcohol users become addicts? Why do so few opiate users become addicts, and why do only a tiny percent of stimulant users become addicts? No one knows! If you could find a difference between the brains of addicts and non-addicts, some physical or chemical or genetic difference, then you might find a way to prevent addiction. Despite over a hundred years of research, no one has been able to find a difference between addict and non-addict brains before addiction sets in.

So how do you design a treatment for the excessive voluntary ingestion of a substance which most of the population uses without ever developing a problem? What is unique about the addict population that they develop a craving which is not true about the rest of the population? The medical profession has no idea. This is not a unique American problem. These same addiction problems and approximate percentages are present in populations throughout the world.

CHAPTER 3

OPIATE ADDICTION AND CONVENTIONAL TREATMENT

Opiates are wonderful natural substances that have been used by humans for thousands of years. The earliest written record of the cultivation of the opium poppy, *Papaver somniferum*, dates from 3400 BCE. The sap of the poppy, called opium, contains morphine as the active ingredient. Morphine relieves a sense of pain, reduces anxiety, suppresses cough and diarrhea, and induces a dreamlike sleep. A world without opiates would be a harsh and painful world! While opiates are not essential for human survival, I would not want to live in a world without opiate pain relief!

Opiates have these interesting effects because they mimic a set of chemicals produced normally in the human body in response to pain and stress. These chemicals are called endorphins. They help us by relieving, to some degree, short-term pain. Your body's release of endorphins is believed to cause the experience of the "runner's high", a feeling similar to a small dose of morphine. Many compulsive runners, if forced to not exercise by injury or circumstance, go through a mild opiate-type withdrawal. They crave to return to running. Nature produces millions of chemicals in plants, and a few of them have the same effect as chemicals in our bodies. Morphine, the active chemical in opium, is one such chemical. The stems and pods of the poppy plant can be crushed, simmered in water and drunk as tea, or the dried sap, called opium, can be eaten or smoked. It was probably not too difficult for our ancestors to discover its properties. Morphine is named after Morpheus, the Greek god of dreams.

Opiate overdoses kill by suppressing the breathing center in the brain. Ingest too much opiate and you stop breathing. More than 3 minutes without breathing generally causes brain damage and in a few more minutes, death. There is a specific very effective treatment for opiate overdose. It is the drug naloxone which kicks the opiate off of the opiate receptor so that the person begins to breathe within seconds and wakes up. Naloxone is available as a nasal spray called Narcan that is sold over the counter in drug stores and can be administered by anyone. Many organizations give away free Narcan Spray to family members and friends of opiate addicts. Generally one spray will revive a person overdosed on morphine or heroin. Sometimes two or more sprays are needed for someone overdosed on fentanyl or nitrazines. It is not possible to harm a person with Narcan even if the person is not breathing for some reason other than an opiate overdose, so when in doubt, give the Narcan spray to the person who is not breathing and is suspected of being an addict.

It is important to understand the difference between the *anesthetic* properties of local and general anesthetics, and the *analgesic* properties of opiates. Anesthetics block the passage of nerve impulses. They prevent the nerve from working. They are temporary poisons which prevent the nerve from transmitting an impulse from a pain receptor to the awareness center in the brain. An opiate analgesic alters the perception of the pain impulse in the brain so that the person is less troubled by the pain. This is a profound difference. An anesthetic can prevent a person from feeling that their finger is being broken. Even large amounts of opiate will not prevent a person from screaming in pain if their finger is broken. An opiate alters the understanding or experience of pain. It does not prevent the feeling of pain.

Aspirin, ibuprofen, acetaminophen (Tylenol) and similar drugs act differently in the body from opiates. They reduce inflammation and affect a minor secondary receptor which reduces mild pain.These substances are much less effective in reducing the pain experience, do not cause tolerance or craving, and have no withdrawal syndrome. They reduce fever, and some of them reduce inflammation, effects that opiates do not have.

Opiate addiction has three major aspects; physical addiction, tolerance and craving. Physical addiction occurs when you use a significant amount of opiate every day, throughout the day for any reason, for 1 to 2 weeks. If you then abruptly stop the opiate, you will have withdrawal symptoms consisting of all or many of the following: anxiety, muscle aches, insomnia, runny nose, sweating, yawning, abdominal cramping, diarrhea, goosebumps, nausea and vomiting. The severity of the withdrawal symptoms will depend on how much opiate you were taking, how often and for how long. Many people who have surgery and need to take opiates for one to several weeks go through opiate withdrawal when they stop the opiate and are unaware that the flu-like symptoms and discomfort experienced for several days is actually opiate withdrawal. A person using large amounts of opiates will have those withdrawal symptoms upon stopping the opiate to such a severe degree that they may wish that they were dead. With short acting opiates like morphine and heroin, the withdrawal syndrome lasts about 4 days. With long acting opiates like methadone, the withdrawal syndrome may last for 2 or 3 weeks.

Regular opiate use for more than a week results in tolerance to the opiate. Tolerance means that to maintain the original effect of the opiate when first taken, one must gradually increase the dose of opiate. Most people who need opiates following surgery are unaware that the opiate is becoming less effective as they continue to take the same dose for several days or weeks. The pain caused by the surgery is decreasing at the same time that the effect of the opiate is decreasing due to the developing tolerance. Therefore, the opiate appears to continue to be just as effective for several days or weeks as it was when first taken. When opiates are prescribed continuously for chronic pain, tolerance is an immense problem because higher and higher doses of the opiate are required to maintain the same level of pain relief as the months pass. Strangely, of all the addictive drugs, only opiates exhibit tolerance as a significant problem.

Craving for opiates is the bugaboo of opiate use. Most people who use opiates short term, for days or a few weeks because of injury or surgery, do not experience craving when they stop the opiate. Even if they go through the withdrawal symptoms upon stopping, they do not have a craving for the opiate. Indeed, most people do not feel good on opiates and will use them even less frequently and for a shorter period of time than their doctor suggests. Many people don't take the opiates prescribed by their doctor at all, or take them only briefly, because the pain is less distressing than the strange mental feeling caused by the opiate. But others, a small percentage who take an opiate for pain or curiosity, find that the opiate makes them feel much better. They may find it distinctly pleasurable. Some of those recognize the danger of that pleasure response and get off the opiate as quickly as possible. Others are unaware of how much better they feel on the opiate until they stop the opiate. Then they experience not only the withdrawal symptoms, but a profound loss of pleasure and a maddening anxiety. A craving for the opiate occurs which, for some people, is irresistible. These are the one percent of Americans who are opiate addicts, about 3 million people. It is from this group that about 80,000 die of overdoses each year. Willpower is a faint shadow compared to the intensity of the craving. It can be so powerful that it overwhelms concern for one's own health and well being, and even obligations to one's own family.

To make it even more complicated and difficult to counter, opiate craving can be triggered by social circumstances. The setting in which an opiate addict acquired or used opiates can trigger severe craving even in a person who has been clean and not using opiates for months or years. Recall that the smell of apple pie can trigger longings of childhood with mother. Likewise, driving by the street corner where heroin was purchased or seeing a fellow user can trigger craving as though one stopped the opiate only yesterday. Many addicts vow upon withdrawal to move to a new town because they have an awareness that the desire to use is triggered by their place of drug use. They are not escaping just from friends who use and their drug dealer, but they also want to escape from the triggering of memories of using as that can induce overwhelming craving.

The complexity of opiate addiction is illustrated by the use of heroin by American soldiers during the Vietnam War. Combat in the jungle, hunting human beings while they hunt you, is a profoundly traumatizing experience generating high levels of anxiety. Millions of pills of amphetamine were distributed to the soldiers by the Army to keep them awake and aggressive. These stimulants also make a person anxious. While anxiety can keep you alert and alive, the daily stress of combat and amphetamine use degrades functioning which can be fatal on the battlefield. Fortunately, the CIA supported the Loatian hill tribes by buying their opium production. They transported it to Thailand where it was processed into heroin. It was flown to Saigon and sold in small glass vials of 1/4 to ½ gram for $1.00 and later $2.00. About 97% pure heroin, the opening of the vial just fit the tip of a burning cigarette. Dip the lit cigarette into the vial, take one or two puffs, and the anxiety cleared without diminishing alertness or cognitive ability. In 1972, 20% of American soldiers in Vietnam were addicted to heroin (defined by experiencing the withdrawal syndrome upon stopping). Before being flown to America at the end of their combat tour, addicted soldiers were held in Vietnam for a week while they went through heroin withdrawal. After the war, a large study of those addicted soldiers found that only 1% continued heroin use in the United States. The others did not have cravings! 1% is the same rate of addiction among males of the same age in the United States who were never in the Army.

The critical value of opiates (and marijuana) in such a stressful setting as war is illustrated by the 1% mental breakdown of combat soldiers in Vietnam where marijuana and heroin were readily available vs the 10% mental breakdown rate of combat soldiers during World War II where opiates and marijuana were not available. Situational addiction is a real phenomena, and is one of the factors driving addiction in the large homeless population in America.

Heroin, fentanyl, nitrazine, codeine, oxycodone etc., are drugs which all do the same thing as morphine. All of them affect the same opiate receptors in the brain, spinal cord and GI tract. They all cause the same side effects like constipation and death from overdose by suppressing the drive to breathe. Different opiates vary in the routes of administration and the length of time that they remain active in the body, but they all have the same actions.

The opium poppy contains codeine in addition to morphine. Codeine is often given to suppress cough or diarrhea and to treat moderate pain because its effects last longer than oral morphine. Yet codeine has no pain relieving properties. Codeine is slowly converted in the human liver into morphine which then relieves pain, suppresses cough and diarrhea. By giving codeine, one can spread out the time that morphine will be released into the body to do its work. There are a few humans that do not have the enzymes necessary to convert codeine into morphine. Those persons receive no pain relief or cough or diarrhea suppression from codeine.

Morphine injected into the human body is half destroyed in 2 to 3 hours by enzymes in the body or excretion in the urine. In

6 hours about ¾ of it is gone, which is why morphine is routinely administered several times a day. Heroin is morphine with a slight chemical change that allows it to move from the blood and into the brain more rapidly than morphine. That makes it about four times as powerful as morphine. Fentanyl is about 50 to 100 times more powerful than heroin and has a half life of about 5 hours. The nitrazines, the most recent additions to the illegal opiate market, are about 10 times as powerful as fentanyl.

Methadone, about 3 times as powerful as morphine, has a half life of about 24 to 36 hours and is typically given once a day. All opiates have the same effect on the brain as morphine. Some are more powerful in that much less is required to have the same effect and some are cleared by the body at different rates. They all cause withdrawal syndrome and tolerance in long term users, but they all cause craving only in some users.

The treatment of opiate addiction, Opiate Use Disorder in medical terminology, follows three very different paths. The traditional treatment is to stop the opiate, treat the physical withdrawal with kindness and if necessary some sedatives, and provide psychotherapy. Psychotherapy means talking with the person about their life and how they might think and behave differently to avoid returning to opiate use. Sometimes withdrawn addicts are encouraged to attend daily or weekly self-help groups like NA (Narcotics Anonymous). The success rate for all of these treatment programs is between 0 and 5%.

The second type of program is to substitute a long-acting opiate, methadone or buprenorphine, for the short-acting opiate they are using and continue this for many months or years. The addict is obviously not off of opiates, but is instead on a legal regular dose of long acting opiate so that obtaining the drug to avoid withdrawal and craving no longer dominates the person's life. These long-acting opiates do not give the sense of pleasure, the high, provided by the shorter-acting opiates. For a small subset of highly motivated addicts, typically well educated and with good job potential, this is quite successful for many years. About 25% of these long term addicts eventually taper off of the long-acting opiate and become drug free. This long-term, long-acting opiate treatment program, however, is helpful for only a tiny fraction of the addict population. The disadvantage to the long-acting substitute treatment with methadone or buprenorphine is that these opiates can easily be diverted into the illegal market. The government therefore maintains such tight control that it is expensive and difficult to provide this treatment to many addicts.

The third type of treatment for opiate addiction is to withdraw from opiates and then, every 4 weeks, take an injection of the drug naltrexone in a long acting formulation. Naltrexone blocks the opiate receptors so that another opiate such as morphine or heroin cannot activate the receptor. The trade name for the long-acting naltrexone is Vivitrol. It was originally designed for the treatment of alcohol dependence (alcoholism), but can be used as a treatment for opiate dependence as well. It does not prevent the craving for opiates that generally drives people back to their use, so its success is quite limited. It has been somewhat effective in highly motivated addicts such as physicians. Those doctors use it as part of a closely monitored program to allow the physician to continue to practice medicine even after they have been identified as opiate addicts. Vivitrol is very expensive and used by few recovering addicts.

Opiate use in chronic pain

Persons with chronic severe pain which is only relieved by opiates face an unending dilemma. If they use the opiate consistently, tolerance develops and it becomes less effective. Ideally, one should use the opiate intermittently in order to reduce the development of tolerance, but it takes enormous self restraint to maintain such a schedule in the face of severe pain. As the patient's pain experience gradually rises as tolerance to the opiate increases, the patients typically pressure their physicians for more and more opiates. This is so unpleasant that many physicians refuse to treat chronic pain patients at all. Those who do treat chronic pain patients typically require the patients to sign contacts, follow rigid schedules of opiate use and require urine testing to assure that the patient is not cheating on the contract. It is frequently an unpleasant experience for both the patient and the physician.

In persons with severe pain associated with a terminal illness, the issue of tolerance is ignored. The amount of opiate is progressively increased as needed to control the pain, there being no top limit for the amount given except that you try not to give so much that the patient stops breathing. The amount of opiate given daily in this circumstance is sometimes truly staggering.

Opiates and stimulants

The pain relieving properties of opiates are enhanced by the simultaneous use of a stimulant. Likewise, the euphoria or high of opiates are enhanced by stimulants. Brompton's cocktail, a mixture of heroin and cocaine, was used in the 1920s at the London hospital of the same name to treat the excruciating pain of cancer metastasized to bone in its first of its kind hospice unit. In the drug culture the mixture of cocaine and heroin is called a speedball. For this reason opiate addictions are frequently intertwined with stimulant addictions.

This combination of an analgesic and stimulant also works for aspirin, ibuprofen and Tylenol. Take them with a cup of coffee for greatest effect. Some over-the-counter headache medications combine ibuprofen and caffeine in the same pill.

CHAPTER 4

STIMULANT ADDICTION AND CONVENTIONAL TREATMENT

Cocaine, like opium, has been known to man for thousands of years. The leaf of the coca bush which contains small amounts of cocaine, chewed slowly, provides increased energy and alertness, allowing a person to work beyond their usual capacity. When the Spanish conquered the Incas in Peru, they were appalled that the Incas chewed coca leaves and considered coca to be a drug of the Devil. They banned its use. The Spanish enslaved the Incas and forced them to dig silver ore at high altitude in the Andes mountains. Their work ability at altitude was very low. This inspired the Spanish to realize that they had been mistaken, and that coca leaves were actually a gift from God. Coca leaves were then provided to the miners so that they could dig silver ore vigorously at high altitude and make the Spanish rich.

Cocaine hydrochloride was first isolated from the coca leaf in 1860. It was soon recognized to be a potent antidepressant and was promoted for that use by Sigmond Freud, the famous inventor of psychoanalysis. The first surgeon at the famous Johns Hopkins Hospital in Baltimore, William Halstead, pioneered cocaine's use as a local anesthetic and also invented rubber surgical gloves. Dr Halstead was addicted to cocaine for much of his medical career. Cocaine is very effective at temporarily blocking the pain receptors on the ends of nerves, but it doesn't block the nerve impulse like other anesthetics. It continues to be used in nasal surgery.

Coca-Cola, the pick me up drink developed in 1886 in Atlanta, combined the coca leaf (a source of cocaine) and the kola nut (a source of caffeine). It proved very popular as it was more alerting and invigorating than coffee or tea. To this day the CocaCola flavor is derived from the coca leaf. In the 1890s, the Sears and Roebuck national catalog offered a syringe and cocaine for $1.50. Cocaine was widely used by laborers and many employers supplied it to their workers to increase productivity. It became increasingly associated with lower class whites and African-Americans, the laboring classes. Lurid tales of superhuman strength and sexual proclivities especially in black men using cocaine led to increasing restrictions on its availability until it was banned except by medical prescription in 1914 with the Harrison Narcotic Act.

Amphetamine was developed in 1910 and along with cocaine was extensively used during World War I to keep soldiers alert and aggressive. How else would you convince thousands of soldiers at dawn to climb out of the muddy trenches and charge machine gun fire to certain death? Amphetamines in one form or another have been used by militaries all over the world ever since. The implication is that millions of people have used amphetamines extensively, repeatedly, off and on for years, and relatively few ever become addicted.

College students famously use amphetamines to cram for exams, and there is extensive research showing that amphetamines can increase concentration and comprehension by about 10%. It is not surprising then that the most effective drug used to treat children with Attention Deficit Hyperactivity Disorder is amphetamine.

Cocaine and amphetamine do the same thing in the central nervous system. They both interfere with the protein that enables neurons to destroy dopamine. This has the effect of increasing the free dopamine in the brain. Dopamine stimulates the receptors on the nerves in the pleasure/euphoria center and increases alertness. Experienced drug users given cocaine and methamphetamine by IV in comparable amounts cannot tell the drugs apart except that the effect of the amphetamine lasts somewhat longer than cocaine. Note that unlike cocaine, amphetamine is not a local anesthetic.

About 4% of American adults, most with the diagnosis of ADHD, fill amphetamine prescriptions and an estimated 2% of adults misuse amphetamines. It is hard to know how many people are addicted to amphetamines and/or cocaine as they frequently are also addicted to alcohol or opiates. Nevertheless there is a distinct and socially disruptive stimulant addiction syndrome. Symptoms include irritability, anger, insomnia, paranoia, delusions of persecution, weight loss, picking at the skin sometimes due to a feeling that there are bugs under the skin, skin lesions, loss of teeth, loss of social relationships and intense craving for the drug. Perhaps surprisingly, there is no withdrawal syndrome for amphetamines or cocaine. Tolerance is either nonexistent or relatively minor. That is, you don't have to constantly increase the dose of cocaine or amphetamine to obtain the same effect. This is obvious in children with Attention Deficit

Hyperactivity Disorder who take the same dose of amphetamine for beneficial effects for years, and do not need to increase the dose to maintain the same effect. It is very unlike the regular use of opiates where tolerance is a terrible problem.

Some stimulant addicts are so paranoid and delusional that they are diagnosed as paranoid schizophrenic if the physician does not learn from a relative about the stimulant addiction. The remarkable paranoia and delusions will disappear without any medication treatment in one to several weeks if the stimulants are stopped. The passage of time without the stimulant will clear all of the syndrome except the intense craving.

Insomnia and appetite suppression/weight loss occurs in nearly everyone using amphetamines/cocaine including children with Attention Deficit Hyperactivity Disorder. Why do some people become cocaine/amphetamine addicts when children are treated for years beneficially, millions use stimulants in combat, and millions use stimulants intermittently for good reasons as well as entertainment and have no craving, no paranoia, no delusions or socially disruptive behavior? Many people use amphetamines/cocaine and alcohol intermittently and never become addicted to either.

Some addicts stop use, that is withdraw, multiple times and quickly return to use. Then for unknown reasons, one time they stop. That does not mean that the craving stopped. Rather, for unknown reasons they became able to resist the craving. There is no way to predict when an addict might reach that stopping point, if ever. So it is worthwhile to withdraw them over and over.

There is much made about different aspects of cocaine hydrochloride which is sold as powder, and cocaine base which is a solid called crack. The practical difference is that regular cocaine can be snorted or dissolved in water and injected, while crack cocaine can be smoked (actually heated until it vaporizes and is then inhaled). Regular powdered cocaine disintegrates before vaporizing when heated and so cannot be smoked. There is no difference in their effects except that caused by the method of ingestion. IV and smoked cocaine reach the brain with equal speed and are indistinguishable. Snorted cocaine is absorbed into the bloodstream more slowly, so the onset of effect is not as rapid.

There are multiple amphetamines sold as Adderall and Dexedrine and a dozen other names as well as methamphetamine which is sold as the prescription drug Desoxyn. An equivalent stimulant, although of a different chemical makeup, is methylphenidate sold as Ritalin and Concerta, and then there is cocaine sold as powder, liquid and rocks. Methamphetamine or meth is much in the news as it is easy and inexpensive to make and therefore the primary amphetamine sold illegally. It is not more addicting than the other amphetamines or cocaine.

Conventional treatment of stimulant addictions is to remove the person from the temptation to use, typically by putting them into a physically restricted place like a rehabilitation facility or a jail. Psychotherapy of various varieties is used in rehabilitation settings and patients are encouraged to participate in self help groups. The problem is that none of this has an effect on craving which is what drives the addict back to stimulant use. The therapy can certainly help the person understand and reorganize their life, but craving can be triggered by merely seeing a drug dealer or watching a movie about drug use. There is some suggestion that one type of psychotherapy, Cognitive Behavioral Therapy, may be more effective than the others in teaching the addict techniques to resist the craving. Therapy does probably marginally improve the quit rate over merely locking the person up for a month or two, but not by much. As with opiates, quit rates are abysmal, certainly under 10%.

In our modern society there are many jobs that require a level of continuous alertness which humans cannot consistently sustain. Stimulants, from coffee and nicotine to cocaine to amphetamines and methylphenidate, have provided the alertness needed to function in an increasingly technical and demanding world, much of which operates 24 hours a day. The most effective alerting agents, especially cocaine and amphetamines, have had bad press for years. In response, the pharmaceutical industry has blessed us with yet another class of stimulant, modafinil, which is just as effective in keeping people awake and motivated. The US Air Force now uses that instead of amphetamines to keep their pilots awake. It has been demonstrated to effectively treat Attention Deficit Hyperactivity Disorder in children. It is still so expensive and restricted in availability that we do not yet know if it will produce a similar syndrome to cocaine/amphetamine addiction and craving.

CHAPTER 5

ALCOHOL ADDICTION AND CONVENTIONAL TREATMENT

Birds too drunk to fly are occasionally found after they have eaten wild fermented fruits. Monkeys, baboons, deer, squirrels, rats, and some insects along with humans will sometimes consume alcohol to the point of drunkenness. Any source of sugar, therefore any fruit, can be fermented to alcohol as the fermentation yeast is ubiquitous and floats about in the air. The earliest evidence of alcohol use by humans was found in clay pots from 9,000 years ago in China. They fermented honey, grapes, rice and millet.

Alcohol is a mild poison, in polite language, a toxin. It interferes with the general functioning of every nerve and to a lesser extent liver and heart cells. This is different from the opiates which affect specific receptors on specific neurons in the brain and spinal cord, but do not damage the nerves. It is also different from the stimulants that increase the amount of dopamine, which then acts on specific receptors on the neurons in the pleasure/activation areas of the brain. Again, no nerves or other tissues are damaged.

To the outside observer, the most obvious effects of alcohol on a person are slurred speech, incoordination, decreased memory and impaired judgment. In the person using alcohol, it decreases social inhibition, decreases anxiety, and induces a mild euphoria. It is much easier to engage others socially, especially strangers, after a couple of drinks of alcohol. An entire social phenomena is built around this, the cocktail party. For about 10% of adults alcohol induces a craving that is difficult to resist. It drives consumption to the point that the person's behavior and social relationships become impaired.

About 40% of adults do not use alcohol, 50% use it intermittently or regularly in moderate amounts, and 10% are addicted and have difficulty controlling their intake. With regular alcohol use, a small amount of physical tolerance develops to alcohol. That is, one can drink a bit more than the sporadic user because the liver becomes more effective at metabolizing alcohol. This is a small effect that does not continue to increase. This tolerance is of a different quality than that experienced with regular opiate use. In addition, regular alcohol drinkers learn to function pretty well in an intoxicated state. This explains why drunken drivers only infrequently have automobile accidents. Some intoxicated persons can drive a car when they can barely walk. That does not mean that they are as safe as sober drivers.

Depending on the length of their alcohol use and the amount that they consume, addicts, those with Alcohol Use Disorder, experience varying degrees of withdrawal severity when they try to stop drinking. Mild withdrawal includes difficulty sleeping, shakiness, anxiety, nausea and headache. The most severe form of withdrawal is called delirium tremens or DTs, and includes hallucinations and seizures. Untreated delirium tremens carry a 15% mortality rate. Modern treatment of alcohol withdrawal with benzodiazepines and the vitamin thiamine prevents virtually all alcohol withdrawal deaths.

Alcoholics in withdrawal should always be treated with the intramuscular injection of the vitamin thiamine. All alcoholics are deficient in this vitamin because alcohol interferes with the absorption of thiamine from the gastrointestinal tract. Thiamine is necessary for normal nerve functioning. If withdrawal symptoms are severe, benzodiazepines are given to suppress agitation, hallucinations and seizures. One might think that the agony of withdrawal would convince an alcoholic to never drink again. Unfortunately, the intense craving for alcohol overwhelms any fear of future agony just as it overwhelms love for family. A non-addict cannot imagine the intensity of the craving.

If heavy drinking persists for years, permanent damage to the nerves of the arms and legs may occur with irreversible pain. The brain shrinks from death of brain cells and intellectual functioning is impaired. For unknown reasons this causes confabulation, the giving of made up answers to any question. Liver cells die and are replaced with scar tissue which is called cirrhosis. Heart muscle may become flabby leading to congestive heart failure. This damage is irreversible. Opiates and stimulants, in contrast, do not directly cause these types of physical problems.

Therapy while a person is in withdrawal from alcohol consists of appropriate physical care. While the withdrawing person may talk and make sense, their short term memory is impaired and they will remember little of any psychotherapy attempted. They are incapable of normal learning for three days to several weeks depending upon the severity of the withdrawal.

There are multiple approaches to helping the alcoholic to refrain from returning to drink. The most frequently used is referral to a self help group, typically Alcoholics Anonymous (AA). In most towns AA meetings are available several times a day and every day of the week. AA operates with the idea that the best way to remain sober is to help others to remain sober. Members are intensively involved in supporting each other to resist the craving to drink. For about 10% of alcoholics this is quite successful. That it costs nothing except time makes it the only treatment available to most Americans. For families with money or good insurance, individual or group psychotherapy is frequently provided, but they do not appear to be any more effective than AA. Note that a tenant of AA is that the craving for alcohol must be actively suppressed for a lifetime.

The medication disulfiram, trade name Antabuse, given daily by mouth, blocks the ability of the liver to metabolize alcohol effectively. This causes the buildup in the body of a chemical that produces nausea, vomiting, headache and flushing of the skin. Some alcoholics use this to try to help themselves quit drinking. Unable to resist drinking even with the threat of being made sick, most alcoholics throw up for a few days and then quit the Antabuse. Judges frequently order legally troubled alcoholics to take Antabuse with third party observation. This is rarely effective as alcoholics generally choose drinking instead of Antabuse and simply don't show up to be observed. Being jailed for defying the order to take Antabuse does not appear to reduce drinking. Some persons from Asia, particularly those of Japanese descent, genetically have little of the enzyme blocked by antabuse so that alcohol consumption makes them sick as if they had taken Antabuse.

An alternative to defying the judge is to take the Antabuse and then drink antiseptic alcohol instead of regular alcohol. Antiseptic alcohol is isopropyl alcohol while liquor store alcohol is ethyl alcohol. Isopropyl alcohol is twice as intoxicating as regular alcohol and does not make you sick if you have taken Antabuse.

Naltrexone, the same medication given to block opiate receptors in opiate addicts, given daily as a 100 mg pill, reduces drinking days and heavy drinking if taken regularly. It blocks the pleasure of drinking and is somewhat sedating. Because addicts crave the pleasurable effects of alcohol, they tend to stop the naltrexone. For that reason, it is available in a long acting injectable form given once a month. That formulation seems to work well in alcoholic physicians who are willing to receive monitored injections to keep their medical license.

The medication, acamprosate, trade name Campral, works much the same as naltrexone in alcoholics. It is somewhat sedating and blocks the pleasure of drinking, While the goal of AA is to help alcoholics to abstain totally from alcohol, Naltrexone and acamprosate are generally given with the goal of helping alcoholics to reduce their drinking.

Fifty years ago many alcohol rehabilitation programs confined the alcoholic in a facility for three months of individual and group psychotherapy. Then studies demonstrated that 1 month of confinement had outcomes just as good as programs lasting 3 months. Subsequent studies demonstrated that 2 weeks of treatment were as good as a full month of treatment. If you have plenty of money there are inpatient rehabilitation programs that will happily keep you for several months. The evidence that these programs are more successful than confinement during withdrawal followed by AA or outpatient psychotherapy is lacking.

While the success rate in treating persons for alcohol dependence is discouragingly low, every once in a while a person stops drinking after multiple rehabilitation tries. This makes it worthwhile to keep trying to help the alcoholic as the alternative is to watch them slowly destroy their lives.

Total prohibition from 1920 to 1933 was a failure at stopping the devastation of alcohol addiction. However making alcohol somewhat expensive with taxes and moderately hard to obtain by restricting hours and places of availability does reduce alcohol behavior problems and deaths. Alcoholics as a group do not drink as much if alcohol is not readily available. The liquor industry, of course, seeks to maximize alcohol availability.

Caffeine and Alcohol

Caffeine partially blocks the unsteadiness and impaired coordination and the sedating effects caused by alcohol. It does not improve judgment or driving responses in intoxicated persons. This combination of caffeine and alcohol causes the alcohol consuming person to underestimate their impairment, and encourages greater alcohol consumption than would have occurred in the absence of caffeine. For this reason the US Food and Drug Administration has banned caffeinated alcoholic drinks. Adding alcohol to caffeinated beverages is now common among young people all over the world.

CHAPTER 6

TOBACCO ADDICTION AND CONVENTIONAL TREATMENT

The tobacco plant, *Nicotiana*, is native to North and South America where it has been cultivated and smoked for at least 3 thousand years. When Europeans first arrived in the Americas, they found ceremonial tobacco use by the Native Americans. Recognizing the alerting and improved concentration provided by tobacco, Europeans quickly exploited the plant by smoking it daily in clay pipes. They added its effects to the mild stimulants coffee and tea which were already in regular use in Europe. Tobacco was soon a major export crop of the Americas.

From 1500 to 1950, tobacco was thought to be as useful and benign as coffee and tea. It was even used by athletes to improve performance. Tobacco smoking received a major boom in popularity in the United States during World War II when three or four cigarettes were included in every C-ration kit, the food boxes given to combat troops. Most soldiers returned from the war addicted to tobacco. Smoking peaked in America in 1954 when 45% of adults regularly smoked. Studies began linking smoking to cancer and heart disease. On January 11, 1964, the Surgeon General, Luther Terry, issued a report saying that the government should do something to reduce tobacco smoking.

The campaign to reduce addiction to tobacco has been remarkably successful and today about 12% of adults smoke daily. Increasing the price through taxation, legally restricting the availability to young people, and a massive effort to make smoking appear as a disgusting habit, have made the campaign against tobacco the only success of the government against any addiction. Note that the government was never foolish enough to make tobacco illegal. While tobacco continues to kill more Americans than any other addiction, approximately 480,000 a year, the number is much lower than it would be without the campaign. The number of smokers is falling as previously addicted smokers die off from cancer, heart disease and old age.

Nicotine is the chemical in tobacco that increases concentration and alertness and decreases appetite and anxiety. It activates a specific nicotine receptor in the brain and alters the nerve function which leads to the beneficial effects. It does not do damage to nerves. As a secondary phenomena, it appears to increase dopamine in the pleasure center of the brain. Nicotine is considered to be the most quickly addicting substance used by humans although not the most difficult to quit.

The most damaging effects of smoking tobacco are due to the byproducts of burning the plant material, not the nicotine. The tar produced by the burning is a strong irritant to lung tissue and this can lead to cancer and emphysema. Nicotine is not benign to the body. It raises blood pressure leading eventually to arteriosclerosis with the consequences of heart attack and stroke. Even secondhand smoke can cause all of these problems which is the reason behind restricting smoking in public spaces.

The tobacco industry has adapted by switching to electric vaping devices to avoid the problem of tar produced by burning tobacco. This reduces the issue of cancer, but does not reduce the problem of nicotine causing high blood pressure, heart attack and stroke.

Smoke, a polite name for air pollution, of any kind is not good for the lungs, whether it be tobacco smoke, scented candle smoke, campfire smoke, automobile or diesel exhaust, oil refineries pollutants, power plant emissions, burning forests or prairies, burning buildings or vaped substances. Vaping is a marketing ploy that puts chemicals and particles into the lungs by heating the substance instead of burning it. The lungs are quite delicate, and irritants of any kind are bad for them including the smoke or vapors of marijuana, crack cocaine and heroin.

For persons addicted to nicotine by smoking tobacco, nicotine containing patches, gum and lozenges can quickly eliminate the harm of inhaling tar, but the harm of the nicotine continues. Social support and psychotherapy of various kinds helps a small number of people stop nicotine in any form. The medication bupropion, trade name Wellbutrin, helps about 20% to quit nicotine. It is interesting that Wellbutrin is an alerting and activating drug sold as an antidepressant. Being mildly activating, it behaves much like chewing coca leaves. The medication varenicline, trade name Chantrix, claims a 30% success rate and works by blocking the sense of pleasure induced by nicotine. Depression and suicide are among its side effects.

The program reducing the smoking rate from 45% to 12% is a resounding success, but it is hard to drive it below the 12%. The addict's pursuit of nicotine does not cause the neglect of jobs and family, disrupt social relationships or legal problems as do the addictions to opiates, cocaine, amphetamines and alcohol. It does endanger the physical health of millions. Conventional approaches to reduce nicotine addiction do not seem to be able to drive the rate any lower.

CHAPTER 7

BARBITURATE, BENZODIAZEPINE, OTHER SEDATING ADDICTIONS AND CONVENTIONAL TREATMENT

Beginning in 1903, barbiturates were introduced as sleeping and anti-anxiety agents. Seconal (secobarbital), Nembutal (pentobarbital), Luminal (phenobarbital) and other barbiturates, were widely prescribed and provided differing lengths of duration of action. Additionally, they are effective in suppressing many kinds of epileptic seizures. Unfortunately, they are very lethal in overdose by suppressing breathing, sometimes addicting if used regularly, and may cause seizures if withdrawn abruptly. The first benzodiazepine, Librium, was introduced in 1960, followed by Valium in 1963. They quickly displaced the barbiturates as they were more effective against anxiety, induced sleep quite well, and were not lethal even in massive overdose.

Physicians had always been concerned about giving a potentially lethal barbiturate to a depressed, anxious, sleepless patient, many of whom had suicidal thoughts and impulses. So when an equally effective and much safer similar medication became available, the use of barbiturates almost disappeared except by states for the purpose of painless executions. Phenobarbital, the longest acting barbiturate, remains in use as there are some types of seizures for which it is the most effective medication. Benzodiazepines also have some minor anti-seizure activity.

Both barbiturates and benzodiazepines act on the GABA receptors in the brain although barbiturates have less specificity. Neither damages nerves or other cells in the body. Both can cause seizures upon abrupt withdrawal after high dose prolonged use, but the problem is more pronounced with the barbiturates. Meprobamate and related drugs have similar properties to the barbiturates and are little used for the same reasons.

While some tolerance develops to benzodiazepines and barbiturates with prolonged use, it is mild and almost unnoticeable. Addicts are generally on a stable dose with little inclination to take more. Social functioning and behavior are generally not adversely affected. Criminal behavior to obtain the drugs is rarely a problem. These drugs are not very socially disruptive.

The conventional method of withdrawal from barbiturates and benzodiazepines is to gradually reduce the dose over several weeks or months. If withdrawn abruptly, significant anxiety, restlessness and sleeplessness occur, and seizures may occur for up to 2 weeks. If withdrawn slowly, the above symptoms are much reduced and seizures do not occur. Addicted persons do not describe themselves as craving the drug. Rather they experience intolerable anxiety and sleeplessness which they know will be relieved by taking the drug. There is a peculiar qualitative difference between the cravings of the addicts of opiates, stimulants, alcohol and nicotine and the desire to relieve the withdrawal symptoms of anxiety for the barbiturates and benzodiazepines.

CHAPTER 8

MARIJUANA ADDICTION AND CONVENTIONAL TREATMENT

The marijuana plant evolved about 28 million years ago on the Eastern Tibetan Plateau. Its cultivation by man is lost in the mists of history. The earliest surviving written reference to marijuana occurs in a book of medicines about 4,800 years old attributed to the Chinese Emperor Ghen Mung. By then, the plant had already been domesticated. That domesticated plant is called *Cannabis sativa* while the wild version is called *Cannabis indica*. Hashish is the dried sap of the plant.

India is the country most associated with cannabis, probably secondary to the belief that Shiva, one of the three primary Hindu gods, used hashish as part of his religious devotion. The Sadhus, devotees of Shiva, give up all worldly possessions and wander about the holy sites of India naked or half dressed, with long hair and beards, frequently smoking hashish and providing irresistible photographic opportunities for anyone visiting the country. While cannabis use is illegal in India and Nepal with a fine and brief imprisonment possible, what fool of a policeman would arrest a holy man or a tourist partaking of the same hashish. It should be noted in passing that the cannabis plant is also used for the production of cloth, paper and rope (hemp).

As with all the other drugs of abuse except alcohol, cannabis activates specific receptors in the human nervous system. These were discovered in the 1980s and are appropriately called cannabinoid receptors. According to the Harvard University health website, the cannabinoid receptors help to regulate learning and memory, emotional processing, sleep, temperature control, pain control, inflammatory and immune responses, and eating. Not surprisingly, cannabis has long been considered a valuable medicine as well as a mechanism of religious devotion and recreational entertainment.

Surveys suggest that about 17% of Americans use cannabis and about 1.7% of Americans are addicted. Relaxation and decreased anxiety, mild euphoria, increased appetite and altered perception of space and time are attractive features of cannabis use along with altered perception of pain. Excessive use is manifested by apathy, inattention and decreased social interest. Cannabis, like alcohol, interferes with the ability to learn. This is particularly concerning in students. Unique among the drugs of abuse, cannabis is stored in the fatty tissues of the body and then slowly released over about 30 days so that one will test positive in the urine for a month after use. Opiates, cocaine and amphetamine are largely cleared from the body in 72 hours while alcohol is cleared in 24 hours. However, the form of cannabis stored in the fatty tissue is inactive on the receptors in the brain, so cannabis levels in the blood are not a good predictor of impairment. This is in contrast to alcohol levels in the blood which are a good predictor of impairment.

Abrupt withdrawal from heavy regular cannabis use may cause anxiety, restlessness, difficulty sleeping, strange dreams, depression and irritability lasting up to a week. These are many of the same symptoms as tobacco withdrawal although the experience is somewhat different. Craving is modest and criminal activity to obtain money to support the habit such as is seen with opiate, cocaine and amphetamine addiction is rare. As with the other drugs made illegal by our politicians, the capitalist impulse to make high profits by engaging in trafficking may implicate cannabis users in crime.

Conventional treatment for cannabis addiction is the usual isolation from the substance by placement in a rehabilitation facility, group therapy and psychotherapy (frequently Cognitive Behavioral Therapy). No medications are known to be helpful.

CHAPTER 9

GAMBLING, FOOD CRAVING AND THE STRANGE RELATIONSHIP TO OTHER ADDICTIONS

In a broad sense, many activities in life involve gambling. A farmer planting a food crop is gambling that the weather will be beneficial and no animal or insects will destroy the produce. Upon eating a new food we are gambling that it will be tasty and beneficial rather than bitter and poisonous. Our brains reward our successful choices by releasing tiny amounts of the feel good chemical dopamine in our brains. This dopamine is also released when we use opiates, cocaine, amphetamines, alcohol and tobacco.

In some unfortunate people, overt acts of gambling release significant amounts of this dopamine chemical. They are prone to become compulsive gamblers. Many people gamble occasionally, for fun or profit, but most people do not enjoy frequent gambling, and only a few, 2.6% of adults in a recent study, are addicted. The gambling addicts behave much like cocaine, methamphetamine, alcohol and opiate addicts. They tend to lose their money, destroy their families and sometimes engage in criminal activity to support their habit.

MRI brain imaging studies show that winning or losing triggers the same lighting up of the pleasure center of the brain with dopamine as does an injection of cocaine, methamphetamine or opiate. Not surprisingly, the conventional treatments for gambling addiction are remarkably similar to those for drugs; isolation in a rehabilitation center, self help group therapy, psychotherapy of various kinds, naltrexone, acamprosate and bupropion. They have the same small percentage success rate that occurs with the drugs of addiction.

In some unfortunate people, the act of eating appears to trigger this same or a similar reward mechanism to an abnormal degree and creates a craving for food that is unknown to the rest of us. This craving for food, especially fats and sugar, may, if not effectively resisted, result in obesity with all its secondary health consequences. Efforts to treat this craving range from taking stimulants, opiates and tobacco which all reduce appetite (food craving) to psychotherapy to self help groups to bariatric (stomach) surgery.

Why on earth would stimulants (cocaine and amphetamines) and tobacco which themselves can cause craving, suppress craving for food? They are widely used for weight loss. Opiates also suppress desire for food without causing nausea. All of them, stimulants, opiates and foods (fats and sugars), can cause the release of the reward chemical dopamine, but two of the three suppress craving for food. Stomach surgery for obesity reduced the physical size of the stomach on the theory that you then could not eat as much. Then it was discovered that just putting a band around the stomach changed the hormone levels and reduced food craving. Now, the anti-diabetic drugs (GLP-1 type drugs) semaglutide and dulaglutide (Ozempic, Wegovy and Trulicity) are approved by the FDA as appetite suppressant treatments. They are stunningly expensive, can have significant side effects such as constipation and nausea, are much more effective than the other treatments, and are safer than surgery. Additionally, in some obese persons who are addicted to alcohol and tobacco, they suppress craving for those substances! In opiate and stimulant addicted rats, they have been demonstrated to stop consumption of those substances.

CHAPTER 10

WHAT HAVE WE LEARNED ABOUT TREATING ADDICTIONS?

1. Addictions are damned tough to treat.
2. They are normal behavior that has gone awry.
3. They affect 1% to 10% of the adult population.
4. They increase with stress (examples are war and economic recessions).
5. Opiates and alcohol have severe withdrawal syndromes.
6. Intense craving for opiates, cocaine, amphetamine, alcohol, nicotine or caffeine drives the addict back to use.
7. Craving can be more powerful than love of family, job and risk of jail.
8. Craving frequently continues for months to years after cessation of use.
9. Isolation and treatment in rehabilitation facilities is expensive and not more effective than other treatments.
10. Family support, self help groups and psychotherapy help a small percentage of addicts.
11. Replacement of short acting opiates with long acting opiates (methadone and buprenorphine) helps to stabilize the lives of a tiny percentage of opiate addicts.

12. Blocking the effects of opiates and alcohol with long acting naltrexone helps a few highly motivated addicts as does acamprosate.

13. Making alcoholics sick with Antabuse (disulfiram) if they drink alcohol is rarely effective.

14. Semaglutide and dulaglutide (GLP-1 type drugs) suppress craving for food and alcohol in obese persons.

15. The missing treatment for opiates, stimulants, alcohol, and nicotine is one that decreases craving, is safe, inexpensive, legal, readily available and doesn't require a prescription.

SECTION 2: PSYCHEDELICS AND THEIR EFFECTS ON ADDICTIONS

CHAPTER 11

THE DISCOVERY THAT SOME PSYCHEDELICS HAVE ANTI ADDICTIVE ACTIONS

In 1947 the Swiss drug company, Sandoz, began distributing LSD to medical scientists in America, Canada and England to try on their patients to see what it would do. The only stipulation was that their results had to be published in scientific journals or reported to Sandoz. Hundreds of studies were conducted and published in the scientific literature about LSD treatment on all sorts of psychiatric disorders. Those studies are available on the internet today. In some studies physicians gave LSD to detoxifying alcoholics and were astounded to observe that the drinking quit rate was about 50% compared to the usual 10%.

Bill Wilson founded Alcoholics Anonymous, AA, in the 1930s as part of his own struggle to maintain sobriety. In the 1950s, he used LSD several times in Los Angeles and found it helpful in relieving his continuing struggle with alcohol craving. He initiated a debate within AA about adding LSD to their program. Using a new drug to treat addiction to the drug alcohol was eventually rejected.

In New York City in 1962, the 19 year old, drug-using hippie, Howard Lotsof, was given ibogaine from the root bark of the Equatorial African Iboga tree, *Tabernanthe iboga,* to try its psychedelic properties. He and his friends found that the ibogaine provided an uninteresting 48 hour psychedelic experience with few hallucinations, but startling other beneficial effects. He observed that at the end of the experience, those who were heroin addicts did not have any withdrawal symptoms despite having used no heroin for 2 days. Further, they did not crave heroin for several days to many weeks/months. He also discovered that ibogaine reset the tolerance to opiates to that of a naive user. It was as if they had not previously used heroin. Lotsof would go on to obtain patents to use ibogaine, the active ingredient in the Iboga root, for the withdrawal and treatment of opiate and other addictions.

In 1970, the United States Food and Drug Administration, the FDA, briefly considered studying the anti-addictive properties of Ibogaine, but was persuaded not to do so by pharmaceutical lobbyists. In 1971, President Nixon began a campaign against many drugs that came to be called the War on Drugs. Along with other substances, psychedelics were declared illegal behind the patently false government claims that they were addictive and of no medical benefit. That ended all legal use and scientific research of these promising anti-addictive substances.

Psychedelics were too interesting and too enlightening for a generation of counter culture enthusiasts, hippies and yippies, Grateful Deadheads, and assorted others to stop using these interesting substances. Smart, sophisticated people, among them Steve Jobs, founder of Apple Computer, Watson and Crick, Nobel laureates for discovering the double helix of DNA, and many other researchers used psychedelics regularly to enhance creativity. A vast amount of knowledge about the psychedelics accumulated through illegal use and informal reporting.

CHAPTER 12

YOU DO NOT NEED TO HALLUCINATE TO EXPERIENCE REDUCED CRAVING FOR ADDICTIVE DRUGS/BEHAVIORS?

Ibogaine was discovered to have anti-addictive properties if persons took large doses while seeking interesting and enlightening hallucinatory experiences. When those large doses benefited addicts, it was thought that large doses were necessary for the anti-addictive benefits, and for many years only large doses of ibogaine were offered to addicts. This model of using large doses, now called flooding doses, is perpetuated by the addiction clinics that sprang up in Mexico, Costa Rica, Portugal, Macedonia and the Caribbean. Expensive 1 or 2 week stays at clinics were only practical if flooding doses were used. No one could take home any ibogaine for lower dose, longer duration treatment without risking arrest upon returning across America's border.

Research in the 1990s which began in the Caribbean and continued for several years in Miami, discovered that noribogaine, a molecule made by the human body from ibogaine, also blocked the withdrawal symptoms from opiates. Further, a similar artificially created molecule called 18-MC had that effect also. Neither noribogaine nor 18-MC appear to cause hallucinations. That is, they are not psychedelics.

Daily low dose ibogaine, 10 mg to 50 mg, causes no hallucinatory effect. After days or a few weeks most addicts lose the sense of craving for the addicting substance. This is experienced as forgetting to take the addicting substance on a regular basis. Flooding (high dose) ibogaine is used to prevent the withdrawal effects of stopping opiates and appears unrelated to the anti-craving effects. Small regular doses of ibogaine also reduce the tolerance to opiates.

Objections to using ibogaine for treating addictions is based on the possibility that it may cause a potentially fatal abnormal heart rhythm in some persons with pre-existing heart disease if they are given flooding (large) doses. The obvious solution to this potential heart effect is to give small doses of ibogaine regularly for an extended time instead of one single large dose.

The GLP-1 type drugs (semaglutide and dulaglutide), trade names Ozempic, Wegovy and Trulicity, suppress craving for alcohol and tobacco, and in rats at least, opiates and stimulants. They have no ability to cause hallucinations.

Extensive illegal use of the psychedelics LSD and psilocybin continued after they were made illegal. Most people seem to have taken them for fun and enlightenment, so full hallucinating doses were the norm. More recently, extensive long term low dose use, so-called microdosing, has been popular for treatment of depression and to increase innovative thinking. There are anecdotal reports that regular low dose use of those substances will reduce or eliminate craving for alcohol, opiates and tobacco. It appears that the doses must be used continuously or intermittently for weeks or months to keep the craving at bay. It is not known for how long this use must be continued. Potentially, it could be indefinitely. Addicted individuals are somehow different from non-addicted people. It is unrealistic to think that a single treatment session of any kind of substance or psychotherapy will permanently eliminate craving consistently in an addicted individual. This is where self help groups or other psychological support as well as continued low dose use of LSD, psilocybin, DMT or similar anti-craving substances is important.

The widely held belief that to be effective, addicts must take a large enough dose of an anti-addictive drug to hallucinate and gain insight into their past trauma or other psychic phenomena is simply not true. Insight gained from psychedelic experiences may indeed help addicts to understand their psychological difficulties, but it is not a factor in the elimination of craving. For example, semaglutide (Ozempic) provides no insight into why a person craves food and alcohol. Yet Ozempic is very effective in reducing weight and stopping alcohol craving in addition to controlling diabetes.

Chapter 13

THE USE OF IBOGAINE TO TREAT OPIATE AND OTHER ADDICTIONS

This chapter describes the use of ibogaine to treat addictions to the opiates, stimulants (cocaine and amphetamines), alcohol, and tobacco. It has been demonstrated to do this very effectively. However, ibogaine is extremely difficult to obtain in the United States. In the next chapter, **Chapter 14**, I will describe the use of voacangine for the same purposes because that substance has much the same effects as ibogaine, is easy to obtain and inexpensive, but has not been as well studied. One must learn from ibogaine and apply the lessons to voacangine. This is unsatisfying, but necessary due to the bizarre and unreasonable legal situation in which we find ourselves at this time of addiction crisis in America

It is illegal to import ibogaine, or any parts of the Iboga tree into the United States. However, it is legal in the state of Colorado to buy, process, possess and use ibogaine and any parts of the Iboaga tree, but not legal to sell it or to give it away! The other psychedelics that have been legal in Colorado since 2022, psilocybin, psilocin, DMT (ayahuasca), and mescaline, can be given away. The restriction on giving away ibogaine is apparently related to the possibility of a heart rhythm disturbance which can occur with flooding (high dose) ibogaine use, that is over 1000 mg in a single dose. This heart rhythm disturbance is now routinely prevented at ibogaine clinics by giving one gram of magnesium sulfate IV in advance of the flooding (high dose) use of ibogaine.

However, if persons are treating themselves at home, then they should not use a single flooding dose of over 1000 mg of ibogaine. Instead, addicts can use a small daily dose, 10 to 50 mg, and gradually reduce their use of the addicting substance as the craving allows. This can be used with opiates, stimulants (cocaine and methamphetamine), alcohol and tobacco. They can use enough of their addicting drug that they do not go into withdrawal. The emphasis is on reducing the craving rather than treating the withdrawal. If after a week there is not a decrease in craving, then the addict is not taking enough. Modestly increase the daily dose of ibogaine.

Note that in France between 1930 and 1960, ibogaine was sold as 8 mg tablets with the recommendation to take it 4 times a day for asthenia and by athletes to improve performance. No deaths or serious problems were reported.

The one danger from this approach involves the problem that the tolerance to opiates is decreased by ibogaine. If the addict uses daily ibogaine and takes their former full dose of opiate to get high, they have the risk of opiate overdose death. This is because ibogaine moves you toward responding to opiates as though you were a naive user. This phenomena does not occur with the other addicting substances.

All of the Colorado legal psychedelics are in the same bizarre situation as marijuana; illegal on a federal level for political, not medical, reasons, but legal in some states and widely used in all states. Users have little risk of legal jeopardy so long as one is not making money by selling them. Despite lurid tales told by the legal and medical authorities, they are extremely safe and not addicting. It is truly weird that the Drug Enforcement Administration claims that the psychedelics are addicting when they are actually effective in treating most drug addictions.

As thousands of people are dying from the effects of addictions which are treatable with inexpensive naturally occurring substances, it is a personal decision as to whether or not it is appropriate to obey the law and not receive the most effective treatment for addictions. Most addicts are risking legal sanctions already because they acquire the addicting substances illegally, so it seems absurd to not use an effective treatment because it is illegal.

In 1885, during the Imperial Age when European countries were conquering and exploiting the resources of Africa and its peoples, the French acquired what is now the independent country of Gabon in the Equatorial Region of West Africa. They learned from the Bwiti People that the root bark of the *Tabernanthe iboga* tree had remarkable properties. Small doses increased hearing, eyesight and physical endurance on long hunting trips in the jungle. The Bwiti had learned of these benefits from the pygmies. In addition, the Bwiti used larger amounts for spiritual experiences and coming of age ceremonies.

In 1930, in France, ibogaine under the trade name Lambarene, was sold in 8 mg tablets for use up to 4 times a day (32 mg total daily dose) to help people recover from debilitating diseases and to counter asthenia, what we would now call chronic depression. Athletes used it to improve performance, just as did the pygmies and Bwiti when they were hunting. There do not seem to be any reports of harmful effects from this type of chronic use which continued from 1930 to 1960. In retrospect, this was the first "microdosing" of a psychedelic substance.

The psychedelics were demonized by the Nixon administration as part of its campaign to suppress dissent about the Vietnam War in the late 1960s. This anti-drug campaign was worldwide and resulted in the banning of psychedelics in most of the countries of the world, especially the First World countries which included France.

Micro doses of ibogaine, 10 to 50 mg/day, may be used to suppress craving for opiates, cocaine, methamphetamine, alcohol and tobacco. This low dose use can also be used to suppress tolerance to opiates in persons with chronic pain - see the last chapter for details.

Still higher doses will be required to suppress the **withdrawal symptoms** from opiates, and because of possible heart rhythm effects should be used under knowledgeable supervision, but not necessarily medical supervision. It is now routine to give magnesium prior to flooding (high dose) ibogaine to prevent the abnormal rhythm (torsades de pointe).

It should be noted that most opiate addicts have withdrawn multiple times either in jail or in rehabilitation. While the withdrawal is extremely unpleasant, it is not what keeps the addict using. It is the craving that drives them back to use. It is the craving which must be suppressed with a substance like ibogaine, LSD, psilocybin, DMT, voacangine and possibly semaglutide (Ozempic and Wegovy) and dulaglutide (Trulicity) or held at bay with social support, psychotherapy or self help groups.

It is important to remember that ibogaine is not magic. It does not work for everyone. No medicine works for everyone. The carefully controlled scientific studies of LSD performed in the 1950s used to treat alcohol dependence showed a success rate of "over 50%", not 100%. We know that there are many failures at clinics using ibogaine. We do not have good scientific studies as to the exact success rate.

CHAPTER 14

THE DIETARY SUPPLEMENT WITH THE ANTI-CRAVING EFFECTS OF IBOGAINE: *VOACANGA AFRICANA* ROOT BARK CONTAINING VOACANGINE

Voacangine is a chemical related to ibogaine which is made by the *Voacanga africana* tree. That tree is closely related to the *Tabernanthe iboga* tree which produces ibogaine. Little attention has been paid to voacangine because ibogaine has dominated the field of addiction withdrawal treatment. The lack of interest in voacangine means that it has remained unregulated and therefore entirely legal to import into the United States. One can buy, sell, process, possess, give away and ingest voacangine, or the *Voacanga africana* root bark containing voacangine, just as you can do the same with peanuts, cinnamon bark, or any other unregulated substance.

The effects of voacangine have **not** been scientifically studied in humans although it has been studied in rats. It has been used by humans with no known harmful effects and has been available over the internet for several years. There are no deaths or adverse events from voacangine reported in the medical literature. Like ibogaine, it reduces or eliminates the craving for opiates and reduces tolerance to opiates. In persons addicted to cocaine and amphetamines, it reduces or eliminates the craving for those drugs. It does not have any beneficial effect on the withdrawal symptoms from alcohol, but once a person has completed withdrawal from alcohol, it does reduce alcohol craving. Tobacco craving is also suppressed. No one has reported the peculiar psychedelic effect that is seen with ibogaine or the vivid hallucinations experienced with LSD, psilocybin, DMT and the other popular psychedelics. That may be because no one is interested in using large doses of voacangine. Voacangine is not a substance of abuse.

The nut of the *Voacanga africana* tree has been used in Europe for decades to make a substance which enhances memory in the elderly called vinpocetine. Because of this, there are hundreds of plantations of the *Voacanga africana* tree in Ghana, Cameroon, Nigeria and Cote d'Ivoire. This makes the root bark of the tree readily available and inexpensive. It can be purchased on the internet on Amazon, Ebay and Etsy. One company from Ghana, ANP Farms, sells it as an anti-craving dietary supplement in three concentrations. Several other companies sell it as the *Voacanga africana* root bark without any efforts to concentrate the voacangine or to determine how much voacangine is in the root bark. It is obviously simpler to rely on the preparations containing known quantities of voacangine rather than guess as to how much active ingredient you are receiving in the crude root preparations. The author has had the 4 preparations of voacangine root bark available on the internet as of March 2024 tested by Drugsdata.org. All contain voacangine and none have adulterants.

The ground-up root bark of the *Voacanga africana* tree in capsules provided by the company Opi-Cure was sold on the internet in 2020 for the purpose of withdrawing addicts from opiates. Because the company included explicit instructions on how to accomplish withdrawal from opiates on their website, the United States Food and Drug Administration determined that they were selling the root bark as an unapproved medication for a specific disease and issued a Cease and Desist letter. That letter is interesting as the FDA describes exactly how the voacangine in the form of *Voacanga africana* root bark was being used to withdraw persons addicted to opiates. As there are no descriptions on the internet by anyone using this technique to withdraw from opiates, it would seem unwise to use it for this purpose except in a controlled and monitored setting. As voacangine is related to ibogaine, there is the possibility that high dose voacangine might cause the same cardiac problem as has been occasionally observed in flooding (high dose) use of ibogaine.

The lesson to be learned is that one must not use voacangine in *Voacanga africana* root bark as a medicine to treat addiction. Instead, one should use the voacangine in the root bark as a supplement to one's diet or to the diet of your family member or friend. As with most dietary issues, the amount and frequency of use determines its effectiveness in improving your health. For most people of normal weight, it is thought that about 60 mg of voacangine daily should be sufficient to gradually suppress craving within a few days to weeks. Do not stop the addicting drug abruptly. Take the voacangine in the root bark regularly and when the craving is relieved, then decrease and subsequently stop the addicting drug. One friend described that he forgot to smoke after being on the voacangine for about 3 weeks. It may be necessary to use this diet continuously to keep the craving at bay, or it may be possible to use this diet intermittently once the craving is suppressed. Eventually, after being off of the drug causing the craving for several months, one would likely be able to stop the voacangine.

Voacangine does not suppress alcohol withdrawal and it should not be used for that purpose. Severe alcohol withdrawal is a potentially life threatening medical issue and should be managed by trained medical personnel. Severe alcohol withdrawal is significantly more dangerous than opiate withdrawal. After the alcohol withdrawal is over from medically supervised withdrawal, the voacangine in the root bark diet may be used to suppress the craving for alcohol. If the alcohol addiction is not severe, then voacangine can be used to suppress the craving for alcohol as the consumption of alcohol is gradually reduced.

Cocaine and amphetamine (including methamphetamine) do not have significant medical withdrawal syndromes. One can use the voacangine in the root bark diet while using cocaine or amphetamine with the expectation that the craving will progressively decrease. The diet can be used in a similar manner with tobacco. There are not as yet any reports as to the diet's usefulness in suppressing gambling addiction. There are a few reports that it may help with marijuana craving.

Ibogaine is not helpful with barbiturate, benzodiazepine or sleeping pill dependence, so one would expect that voacangine would also not be helpful. The literature suggests that ibogaine may even potentiate the adverse effects of barbiturates, so voacangine, being similar, can also be expected to have that adverse effect.

There are no studies of long term use of voacangine in the *Voacanga africana* root bark. Indeed, there are no studies about possible deleterious effects from the long term use of any psychedelic or related compounds. The government has suppressed relevant studies by making scientists fearful for their careers if they study these substances. It is therefore important that citizens who choose to include voacangine or Voacanga africana root bark or any psychedelic in their diet, tell people about their experiences, both good and bad, so that we can all learn of the benefits and dangers.

CHAPTER 15

ADDICTS CAN USE DIET TO CONTROL THEIR CRAVING

All of the potentially addicting drugs provide multiple benefits to humans. Opiates relieve pain, anxiety, cough and diarrhea much more effectively than any other substance. Cocaine and amphetamines provide alertness, increase learning, improve endurance and banish exhaustion better than coffee. Alcohol decreases social anxiety, suppresses cough, is a source of energy, and provides a sense of wellbeing. All of the potentially addicting drugs have forms that are medically and socially helpful and can be legally prescribed.

An addict is a person who overuses substances that the rest of us use episodically for our benefit and sense of well being. Addicts are different from the rest of us. They experience craving for their drug or drugs or behavior in the case of gambling. It is that craving that the rest of us find difficult to understand. It is a sense of need for the substance that in severe form supersedes love of children, spouse, family, job, health, financial stability, friendships, everything that as social beings we hold dear. Whatever the use of the drug has done to the addict's brain, it is so powerful that he/she will sometimes steal their own child's milk money to satisfy the craving. Locking up an addict for weeks, months or years rarely diminishes the craving. Intense social pressure to refrain from the drug is slightly more effective than incarceration as can be seen in the success of AA to help about 10% of alcohol addicts and NA to help about 1% to 5% of opiate and stimulant addicts. Addicts in those programs repeat endlessly, literally for life, that they are one drink of alcohol or one dose of opiate/stimulant away from being a regular user again. The craving has not been abated. It is being held at bay by voluntary intense social pressure.

Little wonder that most addictions are so hard to treat. Most addicts have withdrawn from their drug or drugs of choice multiple times voluntarily, but frequently involuntarily when they could not obtain the drug. The addicts know that stopping the drug to which they are addicted does not solve their problem of intolerable craving.

A different approach, one that appears to have about a 50% success rate, is to use a dietary addition to address craving. Add a natural substance to the diet which will make the addict more like a normal person. Ingest a substance that will allow the addict to use the opiate, cocaine, amphetamine, alcohol or tobacco as needed without triggering an irresistible craving. Simply add some voacangine in the *Voacanga africana* root bark, or some ibogaine, or a psilocybin microdose each day to what one normally eats. It appears that in about 50% of people, the craving dissipates in a week or two. It is unlikely that the craving, if it disappears, will remain gone forever. The addict may need to restart the anti-craving dietary substance or even take it continuously and indefinitely to maintain the state that most of us have enjoyed all of our lives, namely to use or not use those potentially addicting drugs as pleasure calls or necessity dictates. Strange isn't it that in the United States you can be arrested for treating your craving with some of these anti-craving substances as well as for indulging your craving.

Many addicts, if they are able to stop using because the craving abates, may well choose not to tempt fate and so never use their addicting drug again. Certainly it would be a good idea to continue the social support groups like AA and NA, psychotherapy if you can afford it, or other support programs. Remember that addicts are different from the rest of us in that their exposure to opiates, cocaine, amphetamine, alcohol or tobacco has resulted in their abnormal development of irresistible craving. The suggested dietary change is unlikely to be curative. Rather it is somehow a resetting of the appropriate receptors in the brain to a more normal state. We know that the addict is susceptible to those receptors becoming dysregulated with exposure to their addicting drug. So if they don't need their addicting drug, say an opiate for a broken leg, they would probably be wise to avoid it. If they want to use their addicting drug after they no longer crave it, taking the dietary anti-craving substance while using the drug should, in theory, be protective against the craving.

The only disadvantage to using substances other than the voacangine in the *Voacanga africana* root bark, namely psilocybin, DMT (as ayahuasca, snuff or IV), and ibogaine, is that they are illegal in one or another jurisdiction. Colorado has fortunately legalized for personal use psilocybin, DMT, ibogaine and mescaline. Psilocybin is known to work with doses large enough to cause hallucinations, but will also work in some people at lower non-hallucinogenic doses, that is, microdosing. You can grow the mushrooms yourself. DMT is difficult to obtain and to use regularly unless you belong to an ayahuasca church. One can hope that ayahuasca churches will proliferate across the United States. Ibogaine is difficult to source as the producing tree only grows in Equatorial Africa and is illegal to import into the United States. Mescaline is difficult to use because of nausea and relatively long lasting effects.

SECTION 3 THE CONTROL OF CHRONIC PAIN

CHAPTER 16

USE OF VOACANGINE CONTAINING ROOT BARK OR IBOGAINE TO CONTROL/REDUCE OPIATE USE IN PERSONS WITH CHRONIC PAIN

There are millions of unfortunate people who have chronic, severe pain which is adequately relieved only by opiates. Initially, the opiates work marvelously and provide good pain relief. But within a few weeks, the person notices that the opiate dose that provided relief is becoming less effective. To receive the same level of pain relief, the person must increase the dose of the opiate. In another few weeks at that increased dose, the same decrease in effectiveness of the opiate in providing pain relief becomes apparent. This is the phenomenon of opiate tolerance. It is the gradual loss of effectiveness in the pain suppressing benefit of the opiate. It isn't long before the patient and their physician may be at odds over how much opiate the physician will prescribe. Neither patient or physician are being unreasonable. They are trapped by the tolerance which naturally occurs with the chronic use of opiates. Strangely, this tolerance problem only occurs with opiates. It is not true with the other potentially addicting drugs, alcohol, cocaine, amphetamines, tobacco and caffeine.

Ibogaine has been demonstrated to reduce this tolerance to opiates in multiple studies. Indeed, one of the dangers of using ibogaine in flooding (large) doses is that tolerance is reduced within 24 hours to such a degree that the addict is in danger of dying from an overdose if they use their pre-ibogaine amount of opiate! There have been multiple deaths reported in the medical literature from this exact issue - the drop in tolerance occurring immediately after flooding (high dose) treatment with ibogaine.

If ibogaine is used in small doses on a daily basis, it reduces opiate tolerance so that one does not need to increase the dose of opiate over time to maintain adequate pain relief. The person with chronic pain does not lose the pain relieving effect of the opiate even if the opiate is then taken regularly for a prolonged time.

If the pain patient is already on relatively high doses of opiates for pain relief, taking small amounts of ibogaine will modestly reduce the amount of opiate needed for adequate pain relief. Do **not** use a lot of ibogaine or tolerance may be reduced so much that if the usual dose of opiate is taken, respirations could be suppressed.

Voacangine, contained in the root bark of the *Voacanga africana* tree, appears to have similar tolerance-reducing effects as ibogaine. Used as a dietary supplement, amount dependent on the potency of your source, it makes the opiate relieve pain as though the phenomena of tolerance were partially reversed. The perceived effect is that the opiate has returned to a previous level of effectiveness. It is important to understand that neither ibogaine (if you can figure out how to obtain it) nor voacangine provide any pain relief themselves. What they do is to reduce the body's ability to maintain tolerance. They move you in the direction of being a naive, first time, opiate user.

AFTERWORD

These anti-addictive substances are not magic. They, like all other substances used to ameliorate some human problems, will not work in everyone. The scientific studies that are available from the 1950s suggest an addictive drug quit rate of about 50% when flooding (large) doses are used. Hopefully, small dose regular use will be even more successful.

If we lived in a rational political world, these substances would already be widely used to treat craving disorders. Unfortunately, we live in a world where the treatment is as illegal as the addicting drugs themselves. For this reason, I emphasize the use of voacangine, or the root bark of the *Voacanga africana* tree which contains voacangine, because it is legal, inexpensive and safe.

The nut of the *Voacanga africana* tree is used to produce the substance vinpocetine which has been sold and been used across Europe and the United States as a dietary supplement for many years. It is essential that voacangine also be sold and used as a dietary supplement.

About the Author

Charles F Clark lived in Manila, Philippines, prior to starting college at Emory University in Atlanta, Georgia, at the age of 17. Upon arriving at the university campus, he was shocked to discover that he was not permitted to purchase or consume alcohol. That was very foreign to his experiences with alcohol and other substances in Southeast Asia. Indeed, when admitted to medical school at Johns Hopkins University at the age of 20, he was still not legally permitted to purchase or consume alcohol. Most everyone, of course, routinely broke the law.

Now an old man of 84, he continues to marvel at the foolishness of America's efforts to control substances that are socially beneficial and medically useful. That exposure to these substances causes a small percentage of the population to develop an uncontrollable craving is sad. That group needs help in controlling the craving.

Charles Clark was freed from the demands of a medical practice by losing his license due to his whistleblowing exposure of the abuse of psychiatrically ill women in the Colorado Women's Maximum Security Prison. Now, he is devoting his final years to exploring what we might do to assist addicts in controlling their abnormal craving for opiates, cocaine, methamphetamine, alcohol and tobacco.

Made in the USA
Middletown, DE
02 May 2024

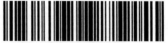

53737650R00053